Fifty Shades
of
Ecstasy

Fifty Shades of Ecstasy

FIFTY SECRET SEX POSITIONS
FOR MIND-BLOWING ORGASMS

MARISA BENNETT

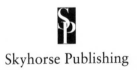

Skyhorse Publishing

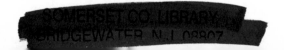

Skyhorse Publishing books may be purchased in bulk at special discounts for sales promotion, corporate gifts, fund-raising, or educational purposes. Special editions can also be created to specifications. For details, contact the Special Sales Department, Skyhorse Publishing, 307 West 36th Street, 11th Floor, New York, NY 10018 or info@skyhorsepublishing.com.

Skyhorse® and Skyhorse Publishing® are registered trademarks of Skyhorse Publishing, Inc.®, a Delaware corporation.

Visit our website at www.skyhorsepublishing.com.

10 9 8 7 6 5 4 3 2 1

Library of Congress Cataloging-in-Publication Data is available on file.

ISBN: 978-1-61608-755-5

Printed in the United States of America

DEDICATION

To Becky and Monica,
who know what I'm talking about.

Contents

INTRODUCTION

Everyone knows how to have sex: Insert tab P into slot V; repeat. While knowing which body part goes where is responsible for human evolution—and by extension, modern technology, telecommunication, great works of art and literature, and the slinky—there's still a little more to sex than just getting it in.

This book shares fifty different ways of doing the dirty, whether you're looking for a few snuggle-savvy tips for being more intimate, simple ways to consummate your lust for each other on unsuspecting pieces of furniture around the house, or how to be the Cirque du Soleil master or mistress of acrobatic sex.

That being said, there is an important disclaimer to this book: Not every position will work for every couple: "But what do you *mean* I can't do a handstand and 69 against a wall?!" cries a slightly miffed and somewhat jilted reader. Well, he's 6'5" and she's 5'1", and that just doesn't work. With that in mind, most of the fun is in using good old-fashioned trial and error to find exciting ways—front ways, back ways, sideways or upside down ways—to keep your blood pumping during each sexy session. Pick and choose which positions you'd like to try out with your partner, or be ambitious and do all fifty in a row (but perhaps not in one sitting—let's not be ridiculous).

This book doesn't claim to reinvent the wheel. Instead, it takes the wheel, looks it up and down, and decides to have sex on it.

Chapter One

Sweet Seductions

INTRODUCTION

While you and your partner may not recite Shakespearean sonnets as you gaze adoringly at one another (or do you?), there's something to be said for the kind of sex that gets you all tingly. After all, it's the reason why people fall in love and (purposely) procreate. These positions cater to when you want to show a little love and affection, lock eyes while you get intimate, or be touching as much of the person as you can possibly manage.

HELLO, I LOVE YOU

Get snuggled up all close and personal for this sweet seductive position. It's a big crowd-pleaser, because the hot hip angle lets him go deep, and sets her up for optimal clitoral stimulation. You both have control over the rhythm and depth of the thrusts, so you can take this position from a slow grind all the way up to a gallop, as your tryst takes off!

He sits in a chair. She sits in his lap, facing him, with her knees bent and placed on either side of his hips. Both partners have a full set of hands free to

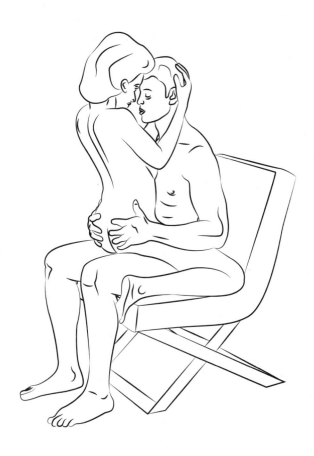

roam around to show just how much they love what they do to each other.

When you're close enough to touch, take advantage of it: let your hands roam and explore your partner. Try touching your partner in new ways: let's be honest, we all tend to follow the same routines, and it's easy to hone into the same hot spots, but when you try this move, let your hands find some new ways to play.

IN THE HOT SEAT

No silly trivia questions for you in this hot seat: just some nice hot loving! Sitting interlocked with your partner, you're on equal footing. This position lets you each take charge controlling the rhythm and speed of your fun; you can even take turns!

He sits on the bed with his legs spread out in front of him. She sits between his legs, facing him, with her knees up and her feet outside of his hips. Both of them lean back on their hands as their eyes meet across the (un)crowded bedroom.

This position has you doing it face to face, but you're just out of reach for (comfortable) kissing. Instead, look your partner in the eye. Keeping eye contact during sex is incredibly intimate; so don't worry if

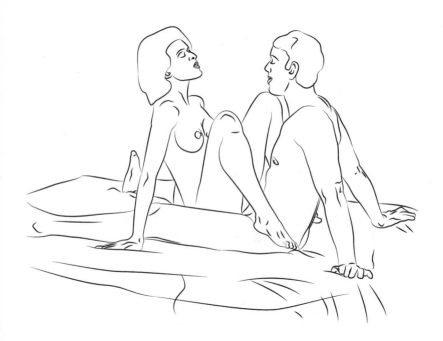

it doesn't come naturally. Watching your partner can be enlightening as you watch their reactions to your movements and touches. We all like to play-act a bit during sexy times, but you'll know your partner is enjoying herself when you can see it plainly on her face!

LOCK AND KEY

He's the key, and she's the lock—it's just one more phallic euphemism, or one more really bad pickup line, for why penises and vaginas should be best friends. But believe me, this is one lock you'll both want to get open.

She lies on her side, top leg bent and rolled down to the mattress in front of her. He positions himself between her legs and enters her, his hands behind her back.

The key's got the easy job here: He has easy access to slide right in. Spending too much time in this position is hard on the lock, and it could cause tension in her back or shoulders, so keep the massage oil handy! Still if you can stick it, this position is a big win. The unusual angle makes all the difference: since with her torso twisted, she's a snug fit! Sideways positions like this one are always good to mix into your repertoire, since they add one more

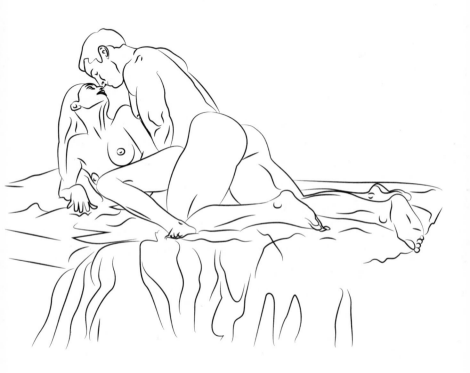

orientation to the "who's on top" question, and they typically give you a tight squeeze.

Sweet Nothings

This position will have you doing it cheek-to-cheek, giving you a chance to whisper sweet words to one another (or naughty instructions!). The close contact and precipitous placement give this position a double-dose of sexy, so you'll be dying to try this one again! Just be careful not to thrust your way off the bed and onto the floor—although I doubt the change in scenery will slow you down . . .

She lies on the bed, with her upper body off the bed supported by her arms (in a push-up stance). He positions himself between her legs, then stretches out on top of her, putting his hands on the floor next to hers. This position works because he supports most of his weight on his own arms, so her rib cage is not squashed beneath him.

For maximum thrusting power, and to keep her from freefalling forward, he may want to press her calves down with his ankles. That way he can brace himself against her for even deeper strokes. She can use her strong upper body to push back against him for double the friction if she wants to get into the fun!

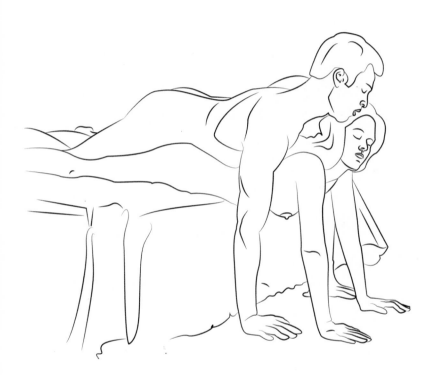

"No, the heart that has truly lov'd never forgets, But as truly loves on to the close; As the sunflower turns on her god when he sets The same look which she turn'd when he rose."

—Thomas Moore

PILLOW TALK DOS
AND DON'TS

B edroom dirty talk is one thing, but what do you say when you want to let your lover know you care? It's all "fuck me!" this and "oh don't stop!" that; what ever happened to a little romance? Here are some basic tips to help you say the right thing.

Do use the pet name you know your partner likes.

"Oh baby, you know I love what you do to me!"

Don't use pet names you just came up with. I know it seemed like a good idea at the time, but . . .

"Oh YES, you're so GOOD my Ass Queen!"

Do give instructions to help them hit the right spot.

"Yes! Touch me there, softer!"

Don't give critiques.

"You really need to tighten up your tongue technique down there, guy!"

Do check in.

"Do you like that, huh, baby?"

Don't zone out.

"Huh? What was that hon, I was watching the weather."

Do try new things.

"Guess what new toy just came in the mail!?"

Don't try new things before talking it over!

"What, you didn't like my new strap-on?"

Do tell him or her what you're planning.

"I'm going to flip you over and ride you until you come!"

Don't talk about weekend plans.

"We need to get the car inspected this weekend, but we can do that on the way to my parents' house . . ."

Stand and Deliver

This move helps you make the fantasy of wild sex-standing-up a bit more doable! With a little leg up from your furniture, and a bit of upper-body strength, you'll be on your way to vertical nirvana. Since your hands will be busy keeping you up, use the rest of your body to control the action. Small movements or adjustments—maybe a tilt of your hips?—can make a big difference in this position.

He stands by the edge of the bed. She wraps her arms around him and lifts her legs to the bed, with one foot on either side of him. He uses one arm to hold her closer to him with the other hand under her thigh to give her a bit more support. She can brace her legs against the bed to raise and lower herself against him (while he tries to stay upright!).

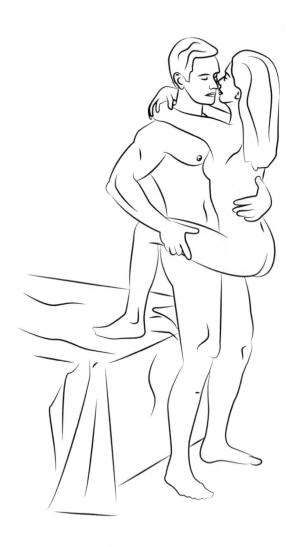

"Then fly betimes,
for only they conquer
love
that run away."

—Thomas Carew

This position makes good use of normal bedroom scenery to get things done! Keep that in mind when you're trying this one out: if your bedroom has a more convenient arrangement, use that to your advantage. Walls can be very helpful here: if your bed is by the wall, you can try this position in the space between the bed and the wall; she still rests her feet on the bed, but he turns to lean her back against the wall. This way he has even more support to hold her up, so they can keep going for longer—and with the extra support, you'll both have better leverage for deeper thrusts that hit just the right spot!

Chapter Two

Doing It with Props

INTRODUCTION

Sex doesn't exist in a vacuum (although that would be awesome). Sometimes you need a leg up, and for that, you need props. But you don't need to run out to your local Kink Mart for angled foam platforms or suspension bondage gear: everything you need to get your groove on is right at home. Knowing this, admit defeat, and just make it your mission to destroy the innocence of all of your household furniture, exercise equipment, and inanimate objects. Now every time you have company over, you and your partner can knowingly smirk about doing it on the coffee table while someone comments on how well it goes with your décor.

BACK SHOW

Sometimes the best entertainment comes straight from your own living room. For the girl who likes it on top, and the guy who likes a nice view of her ass, this hot angle will have you both cheering for an encore.

This position makes her the star of the show and has him as the avid film buff. Like a good voyeur, he

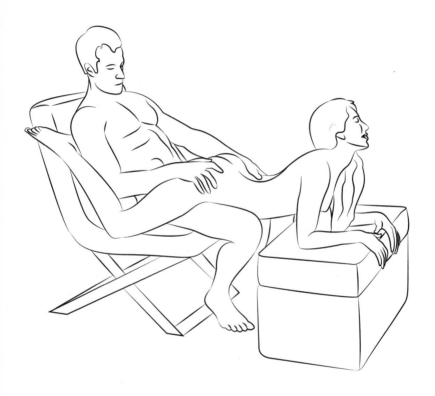

sits back in his chair so he can watch his leading lady straddle him, with her facing away. By leaning forward, bringing her legs back, and stabilizing her arms on an ottoman, coffee table, or chair in front of her, she can control the speed and rhythm while he gets a five-star view of her backside. Managing your props will assist to this end—a close up ottoman will give her more leverage for the feisty and eager sessions, while one positioned farther away will elongate her torso and allow for a slower, more sensual showing.

Just because she's on top doesn't mean she has to do *all* of the work. This angle is perfect for him to guide her hips and thighs as she rides him, or even massage her back. For the man who gets really into his shows, it's also a perfect angle to tug on her hair and grab her ass during all that rising action.

The reverse-cowgirl meets armchair sex; this position features amazing from-behind scenes for any showcase special.

LAP OF LUXURY

Some may call it lavish comfort; others may call it complete laziness—either way, this position combines a good ol' chair sitting with a good ol' sexing.

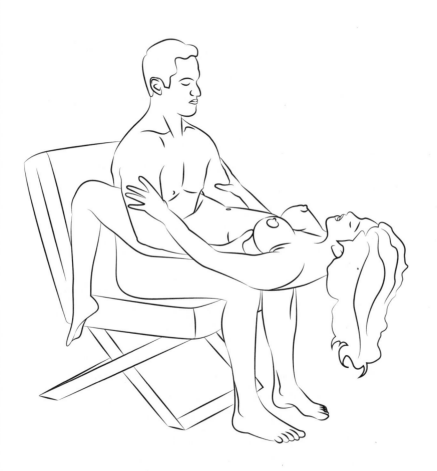

He sits in a chair. (That was difficult.) She straddles him and lies back to rest her back flat on his knees. She should be scooted up nice and close to him, so that not only will there be deep penetration, but her clitoris will get extra stimulation from rubbing up against his lower stomach. This position is the perfect opportunity for him to get all handsy! Two hands on two boobs? One hand on one boob and one hand on her clitoris? The combinations are just so exciting it's tough to know where to start. At some point it might be wise to use a free hand to support her neck—depending on how long his legs are, the position can be straining with nothing to hold her head up.

This position is a great way to sit back, relax, and use those love muscles—so get sitting!

Up on a Pedestal

Whether they admit to it or not, most women want to feel like a little bit of a trophy, and most men want a trophy of their own. This position puts her up on a pedestal, and gives him the grand prize.

She hops up on a table, counter, or high surface. The height of the surface is best determined by how tall he is (if he has to go on his tiptoes or bend down,

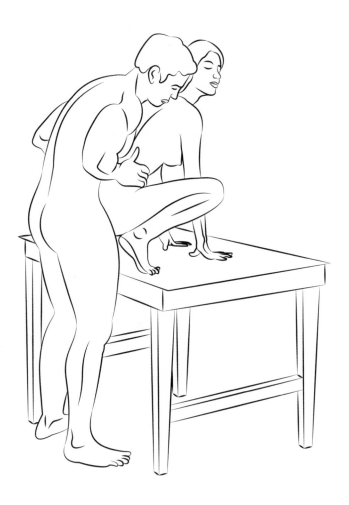

it's probably the wrong height). She should face away, crouching down with her legs splayed wide. She can place her hands in front of her to keep steady. He should be standing up straight, and his pelvis should be at a perfect spooning angle with her bum. (Though instead of spooning, he might want to try inserting his penis.) The high angle of the table she's squatting on will create better vaginal penetration, and give her more momentum each time she comes down on his shaft. Since his stance is pretty basic, he can use his energy to guide her hips up and down, kiss her neck and back, or massage her clitoris and breasts.

This first prize take on a little from-behind loving proves that hard work always pays off.

BALL'S IN YOUR COURT

Sex is a team sport. With the help of an exercise ball and some serious endurance, this position is a real high scorer.

She lays back on the exercise ball, with primarily her head, neck, and upper back supported. As he lifts her hips to his pelvis and holds on to her, she places her feet on a high table, piece of furniture, or wall behind him. The positioning of her feet will give

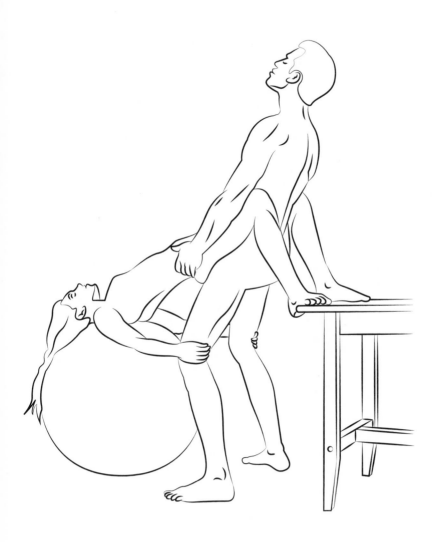

"But pleasures are like poppies spread,
You seize the flower, its bloom is shed; Or like the snow falls in the river, A moment white, then melts for ever."

—Robert Burns

her stability and make it so he's not completely carrying the team, but it will also give her leverage so she can add to all the action. Holding on to his legs will keep their movements in sync, whereas holding on to the exercise ball may have her rolling off court.

As he holds on to her hips and thrusts, she should be using the foot support to do the same! The exercise ball will give a little spring to each lusty bump, sending both players into overtime. Not only is this a fun position to be in, but also it's great to watch! With her lying back on the exercise ball, he gets a full frontal view of her as he brings her into ecstasy.

The trickiest part of this position is getting used to the exercise ball. Just like any other sport, it's important to stay loose and let your body go with it. Once you've mastered not falling off, bring it in for the win!

TIPS FOR USING AN EXERCISE BALL

There's yoga and tai chi, and hot yoga and mixed martial arts, and running on the treadmill; and then there are exercise balls. Even if you hate cardio, aerobics, or generally moving from a seated position, an exercise ball is worth the investment. The point isn't to mimic the exercises they have on the motivational posters at the gym. It's to use sex to *pretend* you intend to do those exercises!

The Logistics

I doubt your local fitness club wants you doing it on their exercise balls (if I'm wrong, can I have their number?), so you're going to have to buy your own if you want to try this out. Luckily they're not too expensive, and you can pick one up at a sports supply store, or just order off the Internet.

When you're making your decision, think about what kind of durability you want from your exercise ball. Most cheap ones are made out of stretchy vinyl or plastic, and if they break, your ass is on the floor. That's less than ideal if you want to use it for bouncy sex for two, so to be safe, think about investing in a "burst proof" ball, especially one made for use in physical therapy. These babies are made so that even if they pop, they take over a minute to deflate completely, giving you plenty of time to dismount before you break anything.

Balancing Act

The biggest challenge to having sex on the balance ball is the balancing! But here's a secret: that's a feature, not a bug! You can use the balance ball the same way you'd use other props like a stool or an ottoman, but the difference is that the ball won't stay where you put it. If you need a little extra stability, push the ball against the wall, or into a corner.

If that doesn't do it for you, you can buy a weighted exercise ball with a sand fill that keeps it in one place. Even with these helpful additions, you still need to concentrate to use the balance ball. You have to pay attention to your body and work to keep your balance. With a partner, you have to be aware of each other's body as you move through the positions, so that you not only stay upright but also correctly entwined. Use the physics of the ball to your advantage: roll with it to add more force to your thrust, and bounce to have him hit the right spot!

Getting Started

Using the exercise ball for sex is a blast, but it takes some getting used to! Start by trying out the basics on the ball to see how it affects your configuration, then work up to more complicated moves. Give your old favorite standby position a whirl and see how the bouncing changes it up. You can even use the ball for extra support for oral positions, rear-entry, just about anything you can imagine, so give it a try!

COUPLE'S SLALOM

Warm up on the slopes with this hot position! Whether you want to hit the bunny hills or go for the black diamond, this downhill take on doggie style brings a whole new sensation to an old standard.

Facing away and down, she rests her hips on the rim of a comfortable chair (or chairlift), while her

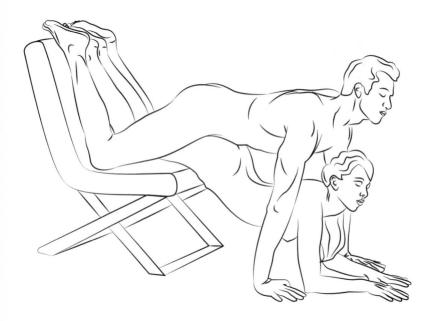

arms support her body in a modified plank position on the ground. Positioning himself directly on top of her, his arms should hover over her shoulders in a push-up stance. Both his and her legs should be casually bent against the back of the chair. This position is naturally upper-body intensive, so the higher the chair or couch is, the more strain there will be. The downward angle of her pelvis will allow him to insert himself from above and behind her, and the sloping position will allow for deeper penetration. This position naturally arches her back, which is super sexy for him, and feels great for her.

Stay on course with this tandem sex scheme and you'll be sure to reach uncharted peaks!

DIRTY DANCING

He takes the lead in this position while she dances along.

Kneeling on a sofa, he carries her in his arms the way Baby carried a watermelon. Her back should be arched over the top of the sofa, while he cradles her lower back and hips against his pelvis. Extended upwards, her legs should comfortably rest against his chest, so that her feet are just above his head.

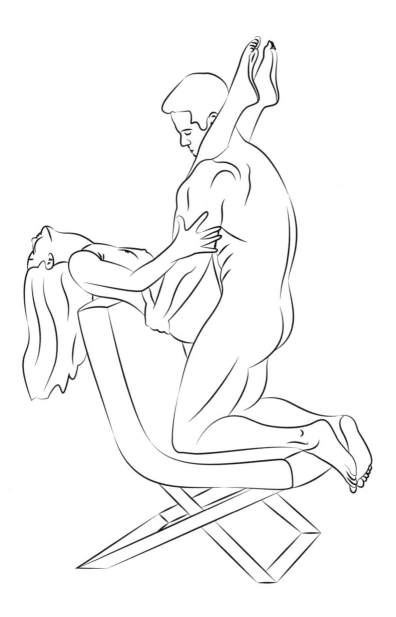

The back of the chair will keep her steady and her hips high so he can use his best thrusting muscles against her. If she holds on tight, he can use a free hand to rub her clitoris, tease her nipples or run his hands through her hair. Keeping her legs straight and together will keep things nice and tight for both partners.

This one is a fun way to perch or be perched on top of the sofa—just make sure you don't tip over.

THE YIN YANG

Taoist philosophy expresses *yīnyáng* as the interconnection of seeming polar opposites. Whether it's dark and light, water and fire, or male and female—one can only exist as long as the other does as well. This position embraces the oneness of two bodies, and the happy circumstance that this unity happens to be in the form of oral sex.

While 69ing can happen almost anywhere, this version is best suited on a comfortable but sturdy chair. He sits upside down in the chair, facing up. His legs should be bent, with his feet resting on the seat back. She hovers over him, straddling just above his head so that he is in range of a nice clitoral makeout sesh, but not so much that he's being completely

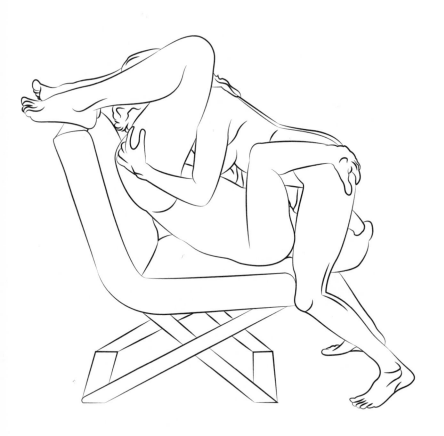

smothered. She should lean over him, hugging his upper thighs to stabilize herself while she performs fellatio. Both partners have free hands for extra stimulation, whether he rubs her clitoris or caresses her bum, or she uses a hand on his shaft or plays with his balls. This angle is easy for her to perform, while the rush of blood to his head will be a whole new sensation for him.

The Yin Yang embrace is an intimate form of 69ing that leaves both partners completely satisfied.

POWERED UP

Since the dawn of earthquakes, fat trimmers, and battery operated anything, vibrations have only meant good things for sex. Whether you purchase a fancy vibrator from a sex shop, or use the hand-held massager you already own for your "back problems," revving up your sex time is sure to send you both quaking.

While vibrators can be used in almost any position, this one is particularly fun for her. He lies down on the bed, and she asserts herself squarely on top of him, facing away. As she rides him, he gets a great view of her ass, and she gets to play with a new toy!

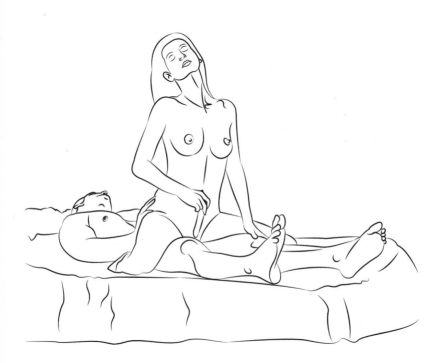

"Let those love now
who never loved before;
Let those who always loved,
now love the more."

—Thomas Parnell

Both partners can take turns stimulating her clitoris with the vibrator—the simultaneous vibration against her lady bits and the feeling of his penis inside her will send her over the edge—probably a couple of times!

Remember to share, though! The vibrator can be just as stimulating for him, whether it's secondhand buzzing as it rubs up against her, or as she presses it lightly against his balls and along his perineum (the space between his scrotum and his back end).

This reverse-cowgirl take on playing with toys is a great way to get you both going. Just make sure to stock up on batteries!

Going Ballistic!

There's something mesmerizing about watching a bouncy ball take off around a room. And like all mesmerizing things, the obvious next step is to try and have sex on it.

He should sit firmly on top of a large exercise ball. Well done! That's the easy part. Whether she starts off with her hands on the ground and extends her legs back, or by straddling him face-out and then rolling forward on to her arms, she should be facing away, cowgirl style, with her hips aimed toward the

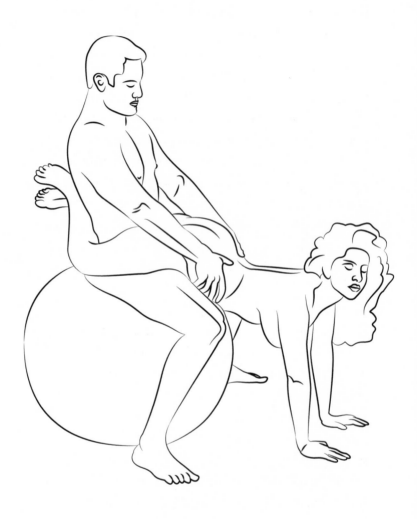

ground. Her palms should rest on the ground so that her stomach is parallel to the floor, and her tush is in prime grasping position in front of him. She should keep her arms straight, but not locked—bouncy sex is all fun and games until someone dislocates an elbow.

Though the exercise ball may seem like an unreliable prop that meanders on its own accord, try and remember Newton's [Sexified] Third Law: Every sexy action has an equal and opposite sexy reaction. In other words, when the ball bounces, those having sex on the ball also bounce. As long as you don't try and fight the direction of all that boinging, this position will have you both springing in the orgasms.

"One kind kiss
before we part,
Drop a tear and bid adieu;
Though we sever, my fond heart
Till we meet
shall pant for you."

—Robert Dodsley

Chapter Three

Old Dog, New Tricks

INTRODUCTION

Rear-entry sex has quite a reputation: like the guy in a leather jacket smoking a butt behind the school, positions like Doggie Style are hot because they feel so *bad*! There's nothing sweet or sensual about it—it's just unadulterated, animalistic sex. There's certainly something to be said for being bad, so why not give it a try? Whether you do it from behind standing up, laying down, or on all fours like Molly the golden retriever, this chapter has plenty of hot rear-entry positions to get your drag-racing motor running.

THE CHARIOT

Brush up on your Greek mythology and make your own Chariot of the Sun. Just don't lose control of it and incur the wrath of thunderbolt-hurling Zeus, because that would suck. This requires quite a bit of upper body strength from both partners, so doing 50 push-ups immediately before starting this position may not be the wisest choice if you want to make it last.

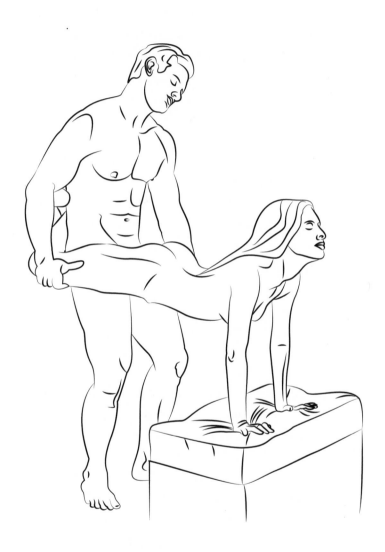

She places her hands flat on a chair, or on the edge of the bed. Whatever piece of furniture is put in front of her, it needs to be sturdy (i.e., make sure it doesn't have wheels, lest she go flying). He stands behind her and slowly lifts her legs to his hips while she supports her upper body in a push-up move. As he enters her, she wraps her legs around his torso for extra stability.

This gravity-defying stunt is hard to pull off, but a thrill if you can get it right! If you have trouble lining everything up, try using different props of varying heights, like a tall chair or a lower bench. Once you've put everything together, you're ready to ride off to the Colosseum together!

Closing the Suitcase

Take the doggie-style position. Now rotate it about 90 degrees counterclockwise, and you get this hot girl-on-top rear-entry position that looks a bit odd, but feels AMAZING! So grab your passport, you've got a first-class ticket on the Orgasm Express!

This spin on the traditional doggie style lets her control the speed and depth of their thrusts while she uses his legs for support. He lies back on a bench or on the edge of the bed and draws his knees up to his

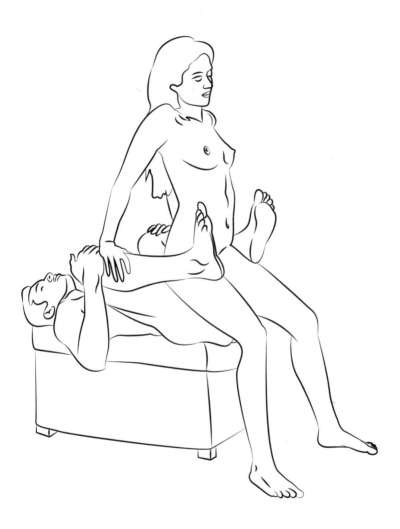

chest. She positions herself between his legs, facing out, as she lowers herself onto him. He can rest his heels on her thighs to help support her and to pull her closer.

It's a tight fit, but it gives you plenty of wiggle room to try different angles and speeds. His bent legs can help her bounce back during vigorous thrusts, and she can rock and gyrate from her perch to create deep new sensations. For bonus points, she can use one free hand to rub her clitoris while he helps support her balance by holding her other free hand or her hip.

LOVE IN BLOOM

You'll be sitting pretty with this flowery position! This move is simple to do, but the twist is in the crisscrossed legs.

He lies on the bed on his back while she climbs on top, facing his feet. She slides onto his penis, and once both partners are comfortable, she lifts and crosses her legs until she is sitting on his hips. He supports her hips with his hands to help her balance. You may have to wiggle around to get to the best position (beware of boney butts and sharp hipbones),

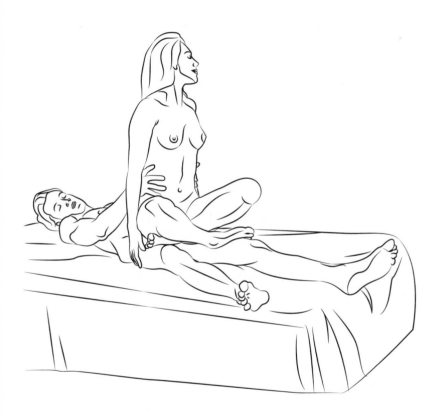

but once in place, the crossed legs give him a tighter fit, and heightens the sensations for both partners!

You won't be getting big deep thrusts with this one: she should control the action by circling and gyrating her hips while he uses his grip on her waist to pull her closer. Meanwhile she can use her free hands to rub her clitoris, or reach down between his legs to rub and fondle his balls. Or she can rest her hands on her knees and chant "OHMM!"

FRONT TO BACK

This booty-bumping position is a more sensual (and prettier!) variation on rear-entry. With your hips resting on the bed, this configuration focuses on long, slow strokes instead of fast, hard strokes with lots of motion. The result is a deliciously slow-burning ride for you both.

She lies face down, propped up on her elbows, with her legs spread. He is in the push-up position behind her, his legs on the inside of hers. As he leans forward, she arches her back, resting her head under his chin. She bends her knees to wrap her legs around his butt. If the angle's not right, putting a pillow beneath her hips will lift her pelvis for better reception. (Getting a penis through the gate is sort of crucial to

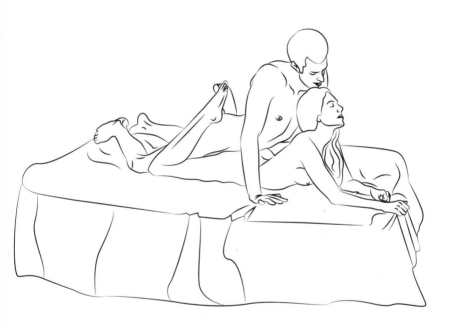

sex in that way, so it's worth being accommodating.) He may be on top, but she also has a say in the thrusting department. She can use her legs around his bum to pull him closer and meet his hips as he moves.

This position gives you lots of room for movement, so make use of it. Tilt your hips (both of you!) for a different vibe, or let your hands roam to spice up this already spicy position!

No Holds Barred

It's no secret I'm a fan of tie-'em-up games, and this position, while silver tie-free, has the perfect amount of rough stuff! Try this position when you're feeling especially naughty.

She kneels on the bed and he kneels behind her. He pushes her shoulders down on the bed while twisting her arm behind her back (Gently: If you dislocate her shoulder, YOU'RE DOING IT WRONG). He then enters her from behind. Even though she looks disarmed, she can still move her hips to meet his thrusts, or use her free hand to give herself even more traction. He can use his grip on her to help him thrust deeper. This position is begging for extras: He can add more rough to the tumble by pulling her hair or swatting her ass, and they both can break out their naughtiest dirty talk.

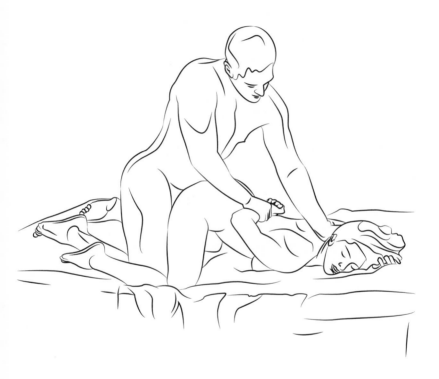

"Touch with thy lips and enkindle. This moon-white delicate body"

—**Sappho,** *One Hundred Lyrics*

A Few Words on BDSM

Having picked up this book, it's more than likely you know what the acronym "BDSM" means. Just in case you need a refresher, it's a condensed set of terms that refers to bondage and discipline, dominance and submission, and sadism and masochism. In other words: fuck me and make it hurt. Exciting sex doesn't have to be rough sex, but rough sex can be really exciting. Here are a few tricks of the trade if you want to play rough, disclaimers, and the occasional reminder not to accidentally put your loved one in the hospital.

Have a Safeword

BDSM is all about sexual experimentation and testing your limits. You and your partner should pick out a safeword, whether it's a color, household item, or inside joke that will be the HALT for when one of you wants to stop. Words that are unrelated to sex are usually your best bet, because screaming, "QWERTY KEYBOARD!" *probably* won't sound like your typical sexy words of encouragement.

Go Shopping Together

Toys, toys, and more toys! A little rough play is nothing without some fun accessories. From massage oils to spanking skirts to floggers and paddles, there are endless options for incorporating inanimate objects into your love sessions. Going to a sex shop or looking online is also a great thing to do as a couple. It's a fun way to suggest things you wouldn't normally bring up: "Ha! Honey, look! It's a build-your-own sex swing kit! How hilarious! Can you imagine?! But, but really—if you want it . . . "

Trade Roles

Generally speaking, in BDSM play there is a dominant partner and a submissive partner. The flogger and the floggee, the professor and the pupil, the librarian and the truant book-borrower—you get the point. Both roles can be incredibly fun (there is no wrong end of a sexy spanking), but it's even more fun to switch things up a bit. Just because he likes to pull her hair doesn't mean he's against being handcuffed to the bed!

Abuse and BDSM are NOT Two Sides of the Same Coin

Now that BDSM has hit mainstream media, it has become a hot button issue about whether incorporating bondage, pain play, or roughness into your sex life is unhealthy or abusive. BDSM can range from experimentation with spanking to an entire domination and submission lifestyle as a couple.

Healthy couples discuss their sexual preferences with one another, and draw lines in the sand about what is okay and what is not okay. Some people like to get spanked during sex, some like to be tied up, and some want to get hit with a riding crop. It's not for everyone, but it is also NOT the same as being abused by your partner. Taking real-life issues out during sex—whether verbally or physically—is completely inappropriate. Please, please note—if you are worried your relationship is abusive, it probably is. You should never stay in a scenario where you feel unsafe.

LAID OUT

This position looks complicated, but if you take your time and move into it in steps, you'll have no trouble with it! This neat rear-entry has a feature that you often miss banging from behind: some love for the clitoris. When she bends forward, she's not just giving him a fantastic view of her ass; she's also tilting her body so that each thrust rubs her the right way.

He sits on the bed with his legs straight out in front of him. She sits on his lap with her knees outside his legs, her back against his chest, as she slides him inside of her. Once he's in position, she leans forward toward his legs as he helps tuck her legs behind him. She slowly stretches further until she is laying face down between his outstretched legs. Her hips

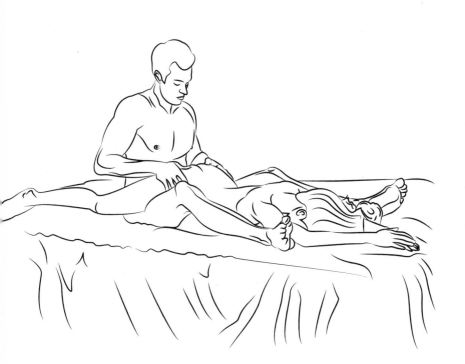

should be up a bit, resting on his thighs, to help get the right thrusting angle. She can grab his ankles for leverage while he holds on to her hips.

RUNNING START

You'll be on the blocks constantly once you master this position. It's a hot mix of tight fit, nice view, and easy assembly, so it's a shoe-in for the gold ribbon! Try this out if you're feeling pseudo-athletic, and it will make you feel like a true Olympian!

She crouches on the bed in the runner's position, with one leg bent into a lunge and the other stretched straight back. He positions himself between her legs, straddling the outstretched leg, and kneels behind her. She supports her weight on her elbows.

Here he's got plenty of room for movement, and her back leg-front leg position makes it an extra tight squeeze. She can always switch legs if she gets tired. If she can balance it, she can use a free hand for some manual stimulation, or he can reach under her bent leg and give her a hand of his own.

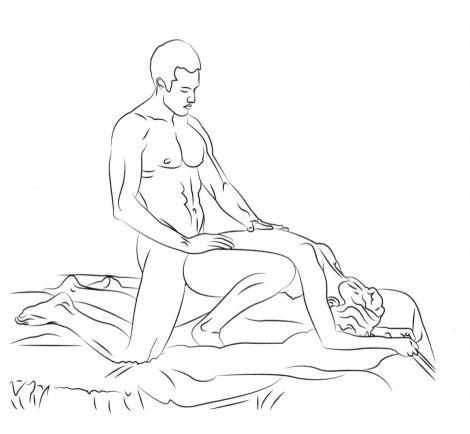

THE MERMAID

This position is a hot way to get tail—even though you need legs to make it work. You need a bit of balance to pull this move off, but it's still pretty simple (and kind of pretty!).

He sits in a big chair. She sits on his lap facing his feet, and slides onto his penis. She tucks her legs on either side of the chair as she slowly leans forward, resting her hands on his thighs. She arches her back to intensify the move.

This move is a great rear-entry position with a tight fit! The tilt of her hips gives this one a different kind of feel, and she can try leaning forward more and more to change the sensations. The more she bends, the more access he has to squeeze, smack, or fondle her ass.

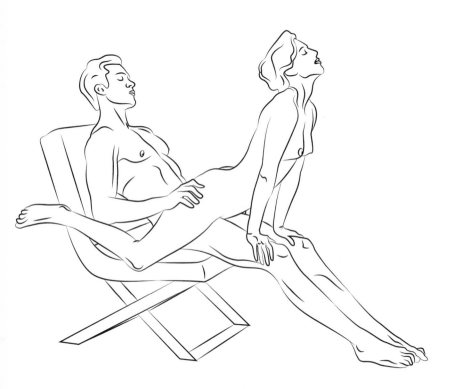

"At such a time she should take hold of her lover by the hair, and bend his head down, and kiss his lower lip, and then, being intoxicated with love, she should shut her eyes and bite him in various places."

—*The Kama Sutra*

Chapter Four

Twisted Trysts

Introduction

*I*f you put your leg on the blue dot, and I put *mine on the yellow* . . . Trying to have sex like you're competing for a Twister championship can get a little tricky. Thankfully, it usually pays off, whether because you've managed to find the right combination of flailing legs and arms, or because screwing it up and falling off the bed is just as fun as being a sommelier of bendy sex. These moves are all twisty fun, so get in touch with your inner salted pretzel and try out these tantric tangles.

All Tangled Up

Like vines of ivy winding along a brick wall, this position makes it difficult to tell where one ends and the other begins.

This position is most easily begun in a spooning position, with her being the little spoon. She should turn to lay mostly flat on her back, while he brings his upper leg in between hers. Her upper leg should be lifted to give enough space for him to insert him-

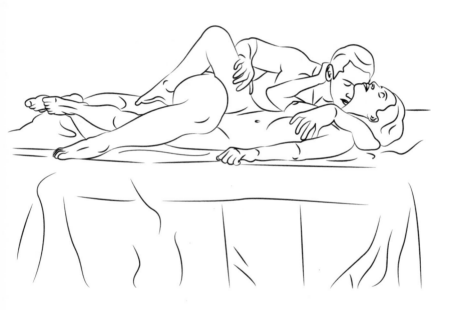

self from behind, and her knees should be bent over his leg so that she can use it to help her thrust. Their intertwining legs will make for a slower, more sensual pace where both partners can glide along each other. Since her upper body is still laying flat, he can still lean in and nibble at her ears, kiss her neck, or move in for a steamy make out. He can use his upper arm to linger a soft hand along her legs, tease her clitoris, or hold on to her hips. In the meantime, his lower arm can be under her to support her head, and the free hand is in perfect range to cup and massage her breast.

Get all tangled up with your partner, whether it's in the sheets, or in a patch of ivy (just make sure it's not poisoned).

PIN–UP GIRL

Half the fun of sex is being able to watch how sexy your partner looks while you get down and dirty with each other. This position has her demurely poised for him, for that classically sexy look of the pin-up generation.

No acrobatics required! This one has her lying down on the bed, floor, or basically any other surface

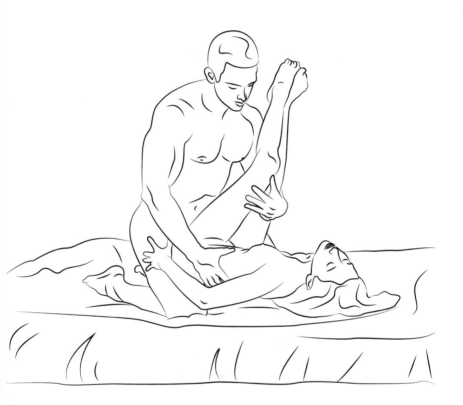

you don't mind having sex on. He kneels in front of her, while she scoots her butt to meet him. Both of her legs should be raised, but this one isn't a flexibility contest. Her legs can be bent comfortably, and pivoted slightly to one side so they rest on his shoulder. He can support her legs with one hand, while he guides her hips with the other. This position has her lying comfortably out on the bed, which will give him access to her breasts, and the ability to gauge her facial expressions (otherwise known as her I'm-Almost-There! -O-Meter). Keeping her legs together will make it a nice, tight fit, and the angle of her raised hips will bring him deeper inside her.

This position is incredibly easy, but a classic for a reason!

SHIPS PASSING IN THE NIGHT

Not every position has to feel like only a contortionist could do it. For those of us who like to try out new angles—hold the torn ligament—this one is just right.

Both partners should lie down on the bed parallel to one another, facing the same side of the room. His head should be at her feet, and her feet should

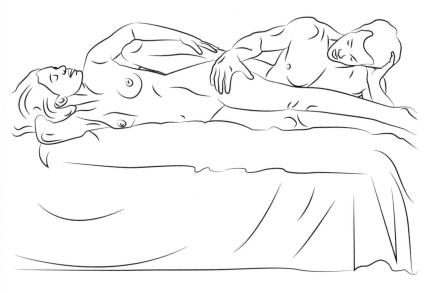

be at his head. He should enter her from behind, and if necessary, her body can be angled in a slight L in order to let him in more easily. This position isn't the crazy-sex-hair-giving kind. It mostly stays at a slow, sensual pace, where both partners can caress and tease one another, working up to a slow, long climax. He can tease her clitoris, and she can reach a hand between his legs to massage his balls.

Be careful not to get too comfy, though—nobody likes it when a partner falls asleep on the job!

REVERSE COWBOY

Everyone knows how much fun reverse cowgirl can be, but what about a little reverse action for him? This position puts him in charge of the lasso and her who gets taken for a ride.

This one requires some furniture that can handle a good romp. It works best with a comfortable chair and an ottoman, but can be substituted with a couch. Since this position is a little nontraditional, he may not be used to putting his penis in from upside down. Giving her some warm-up cunnilingus or sensual foreplay will make it a lot easier for him to slip in when it's time to get rolling. She should sit

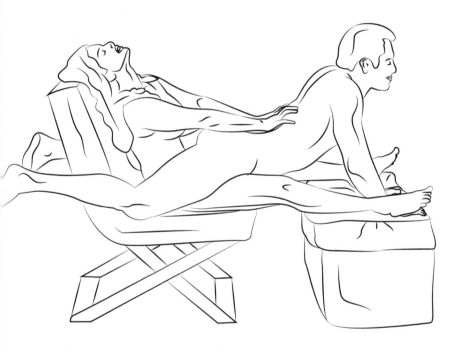

back in her favorite chair, with her legs extended onto the ottoman in front of her. He should straddle her, facing away, using the ottoman in front of him for support. The chair works best here so that his legs can lie flat behind it, whereas with a couch he'll have to bend his legs up and have less space to move. The tricky part is making the entrance. She should keep her legs wide while he faces his pelvis down and forward while he goes in. Once this has happened, it's a lot easier to keep in sync. She gets a rarely seen view of his butt, and he gets to feel her from a whole new angle.

JIGSAW PUZZLE

Putting together a puzzle on a rainy day is a great way to keep your mind sharp. But for sunny days, hazy days, or days that end in Y, putting together those penis and vagina puzzles keeps everything else sharp.

She lies down perpendicularly across a chair. She should bring her knees to her chest to make room for him to join the puzzle. From there, he should squat down, facing away, and angle his hips forward so that he can enter her from above. She can rest her

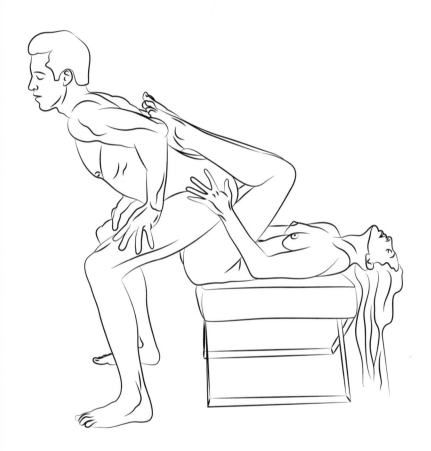

legs on his back, which is a convenient lounging position for her, and will also keep things nice and tight for him. This position is particularly fun, because, hey! His penis is upside down! The flip-flopping of sexy parts will give attention to all sorts of sensitive zones that traditional sex doesn't usually hit. Because of the angle, he'll also surprise her with a steady rhythm of pressure from his balls on her clitoris as he pumps away.

Adding a little human Tetris to your repertoire is the best way to figure out how you fit together!

MODERN DANCE

You don't need a background in ballet to make your sexy sessions look like Swan Lake. With a little upper body strength from him, and some leg extensions from her, your next rendezvous will be the best choreography yet!

She should lie on her side on the edge of the bed, so that her hips come to the edge. He stands at the edge of the bed, facing forward. After she straightens her leg so that her toes point to the ceiling, he should take hold of her thigh, and bring it close to his chest so that her leg extends beyond his shoul-

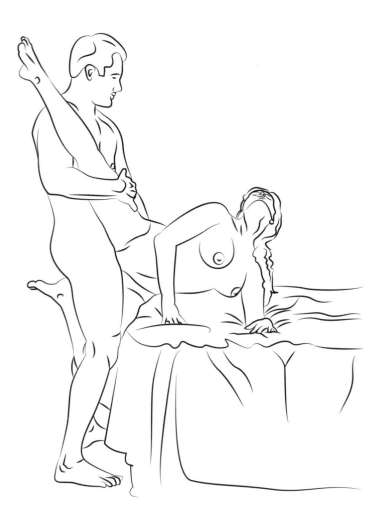

ders. With his other hand, he can support her bum or hips. She should use her elbow to keep her torso lifted off the bed. Her other leg should be comfortably folded in between his legs. She should use her arms to push up from the bed every time he pulls her up in a lusty thrust.

This position requires a lot of upper body strength from both partners, but is worth it because of how deeply he can penetrate her, and because it explores the highly underrated sideways entrance.

The Turntable

There's a little bit of a DJ in all of us. Whether you want to do the spinning, or you want your record spun, this hot take on sideways loving will give your trysts a new remix.

She lies down on the bed, bringing her knees to her chest. Her feet should be up in the air, but they don't need to be spread far apart. Instead of lying directly on top of her, he should angle himself perpendicularly over her. Entering her sideways gives both of them a tight squeeze and she can make him even more snug inside by tightening her thighs together.

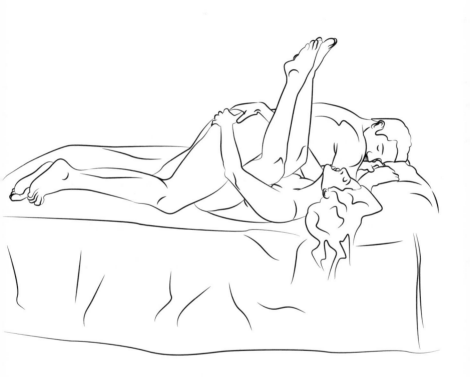

She can continue to alter the sensations by leaning her closed legs to one side or another.

This position gives him creative control over the pace and rhythm of the encounter, while she gets to lie back and feel him work.

PRIM AND PROPER

A good girl should always keep her legs crossed. This position lets her be a good girl while she does bad girl things!

She lies down on the bed, with him on his knees directly in front of her. She should cross her legs so that her right foot rests on his right shoulder, and her left foot rests on his left shoulder. He can hold on to either her ankles or knees to keep her in place. She can cross her legs by her shins, or for a tighter fit, cross above the knee. Changing where her legs are crossed throughout this lusty session will keep things interesting. This is a great angle for both partners to watch each other work as things get steamy.

Though he is in the most control in this position, she doesn't have to just lay back and hang out. She can squeeze her PC muscles to help make a pulsing,

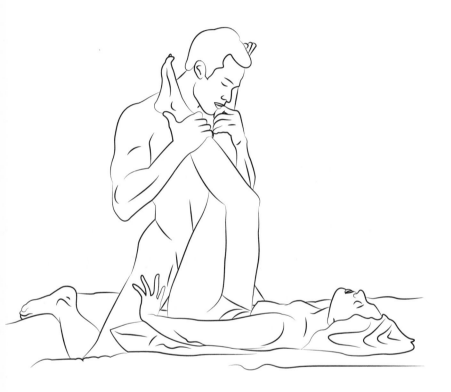

"Thus if men and women act according to each other's liking, their love for each other will not be lessened even in one hundred years."

—*The Kama Sutra*

"Ye Gods! annihilate
but space and time,
And make two lovers
happy."

—Alexander Pope

tighter sensation around his shaft, or if she wants to give him a good show, tease her own nipples and squeeze her breasts every time his motions have made an especially good impact!

IS THAT YOUR LEG OR MINE?

There are some positions that you try because you're feeling acrobatic, some because of yoga, and others that happen because in all that rolling around, you've managed to get tangled into one big, sensational feeling jumble. This is one of those!

He lies down on the bed with his knees up and feet raised slightly in the air. She faces away, crouching down over his pelvis with her feet flat on the bed and her knees up. Instead of keeping both of her feet in between his legs, she should have one leg between his legs, and the other straddled over his right leg (or left, if she's a lefty). Her hips should face the thigh she is straddling. Because his legs are perched a little bit off the bed, his upper thigh will graze her clitoris as she takes the reins of this twisty dynamic. He has free hands to fondle as he pleases, while she can use her hands to either guide herself up and down, or cup and massage his balls as she goes.

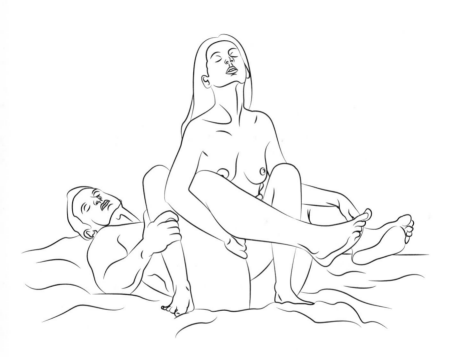

In this leggy tryst, she's in the captain's chair. The angle of both partners' hips is perfect for extra deep penetration, and his tangled legs against her sensitive spots will keep her dedicated to getting him there.

NAUGHTY ROLL-UP

If regular 69ing has got you down (since, you know, being upside down on someone while you simultaneously perform and receive mind-blowing head is so boring), try out the naughty version!

This one requires a little bit of flexibility from her, so make sure she stretches first! She lies down on the bed, and raises her legs in the air, as parallel to her own head as possible. If she can clasp on to her ankles with straightened legs, woohoo! If not, she's like the other 90 percent of the population without a PhD in Being Bendy, and that's totally fine. Holding on to the back of her knees works too. He should kneel over her, so that his penis is accessible to her mouth without her having to do much of anything. With his arms on either side of her hips, or grasping her bum, he should be face to face with her sweet spot.

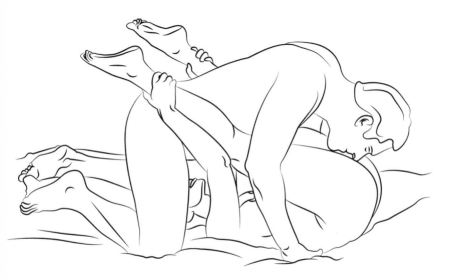

This is where roads diverge. This position is spectacular for giving and receiving some good old-fashioned fellatio, but it also gives the opportunity for some backdoor attention. If you and your partner are comfortable, try letting your tongue explore some new places. Your front end isn't the only place packed with nerves ready to be teased! If not, being curled up in a ball while you 69 is still pretty effing sexy. Everyone wins!

Be forward thinking and try out this role-reversal!

GETTING CHEEKY: BEGINNER'S BUTT SEX

Sex can be weird. Everybody has their own thing that they are into, and anal sex is one of those things that you are just into, or not. But whether you're an old pro or more of a backdoor beginner, these tips will help you make the best of your anal experience!

Only If You Want To

Butt sex is THE WORST if you're really not into it. If you're nervous or scared, you tense up, and your butt locks down like Fort Knox. Obviously you have to relax, and you have to do that by making anal sex as un-stressful (and fun) as possible!

Start Small

Dildos, vegetables, penises, and other sizable objects are bad choices for your first anal play sessions. Instead, start small, using just your fingers. You can also find small sex toys intended for first time anal play any-where fine sex toys are sold; but if you're playing with a real beginner, be advised that if you come at them with something called a "butt plug" or anything rubbery and blue, you might get a black eye instead of a good time! Toys can be fun, but make sure every-one's on board before anything goes in the bum!

Use Lube

Oh God, so much lube. This is the main secret to good butt sex: You don't want friction when you're doing the backdoor tango, and since there's no natural ass lubrication, you're going to want to get your hands on some lube. The last thing you want when you're just starting out with anal is a dry bum, so lube it up before you get started.

Take It Slow

The first time you try anal sex, it's best to take it in stages. Start by getting used to the feeling of having your ass touched: you (or your partner) rub around the outside of your asshole, gently spreading lube around. Once that feels good, you can start thinking about insertion. It's best to let the owner of the ass control how and when that happens, so a good trick for a first timer is to leave whatever you're inserting stationary, and give the butt-sexed partner plenty of room to impale themselves. If you're trying anal sex that involves a real live penis, you want to be extra careful starting out. Remember to let the owner of the ass control the action, which means that there should be no thrusting or movement until she (or he) says so! Butts are great, and anal sex is widely enjoyed, but it has to be something enjoyed by all parties, and not something to check off a list of "sex things I do." A lot of times when couples try anal sex it's more about the idea and the imagery, and all the sexy things that go along with "butt stuff." If you actually want to add anal play to your bedroom repertoire, make sure it is because you both like what you're doing!

Say Thank You!

Make sure you tell your partner how great they are. This is always a good idea, but when you're trying new things and being adventurous in the bedroom, it's especially important to take time to let your partner know how much they turn you on, and how much you enjoyed your sexy times. Because everyone likes to be appreciated! So if your partner is open to letting you put things up his or her butt, make sure you let them know that you appreciate it.

Chapter Five

Deep Impact

INTRODUCTION

Having deep, penetrating sex should not be taken lightly. It has been passed down by our forefathers, the Romans, or maybe Australopithecus—not because it changes the mathematics of sex (P+V = O), but because it feels fucking phenomenal. Skip the shallow end and dive right into subterranean waters with these deeply moving angles.

OPENING NIGHT

Private showings are always the best showings. This position's debut is sure to be an instant success.

Lying on the bed, she should spread her legs for him to enter her. And you're done.

I kid, I kid! There's more! With the help of a little daily stretching, she should splay her legs in the air into a wide split. Straightening her legs all the way is more for fashion than function, so if she's not super duper flexible, fret not! (No one expects him to be an acrobat, so she shouldn't lose points for that

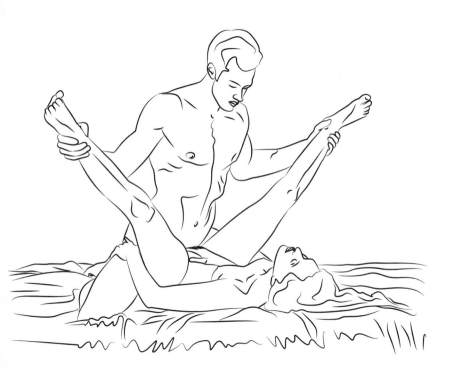

"O Love, O fire! once he drew With one long kiss my whole soul through My lips, as sunlight drinketh dew."

—Alfred Tennyson

either!) Depending on said bendiness, he should keep her legs apart by holding on to her either ankles (for a wide split) or her knees (for a thinner split).

While he works hard in between her legs, she can pleasure herself. Some women worry that masturbating during sex will make him think she prefers her own hand to his penis. Au contraire: "I was so aroused with your penis inside me that I just had to touch myself," should never be interpreted as anything other than an enormous ego boost to him. Touch away.

Naturally, this position is an aesthetic A+, but it also lets both partners get deeply acquainted!

FIFTY BEAUTIFUL EUPHEMISMS FOR LADY SELF-LOVIN'

Everybody needs a little magic touch once in a while. While it might seem like a dude-dominated sport, it shouldn't be news that ladies like a little self-love once in a while. There are plenty of fun phrases guys can use to describe their time spent flying solo, but I have always been disappointed at the lack of creative terms for lady masturbation. But no more! Forget about "flicking the bean" and scrub "petting the beaver" from your brain, and enjoy these 50 lovely euphemisms for sex with the one you love most.

Gilding the Lily
Bopshebopping
Spinning the dial
Dialing the Rotary
    Phone
Hitchhiking South
Riding the Unicycle
Ménage a Moi
Pressing your Pleats
Fiddling your Diddle
Finger Dancing
Doing it in the
    French Way
Tending the Secret
    Garden
Slapping the Bass
Smacking the Pony

Riding the Unicorn
Kickin' it with BOB
Groping the Grotto
Shooting the Pink
    Marble
Trolling the Bermu-
    da Triangle
Beating around the
    Bush
Buffing the Jewel
Reading in Braille
Spanking Lucy
Pat the Bunny
5 Digit Disco
Double-Clicking the
    Mouse
Playing Poker

Manual Override	The Virgin's Release
Twiddle the Fiddle	Nulling the Void
Finger Banging	Hula-hooping
Playing Pianist	Romancing Thy
Falling Down the	Own
Rabbit Hole	The Record Scratch
To Pluck One's	Exploring the Deep
Twanger	South
Tiptoeing through	Parting the Petals
the Tulips	Night In with the
Paddling the Canoe	Girls
Strip Mining	Playing Solitaire
Pushing your Own	Ringing the Doorbell
Buttons	Sending a Telegram
Strumming the Banjo	Jilling Off

TOUCHDOWN

The position for all those who are footloose and fan-cy-free. In other words, it works for anyone ranging from the foot fetishist to those not totally grossed out by being near feet.

She lies on her back with her knees hugged to her chest. He kneels in front of her where he's most com-

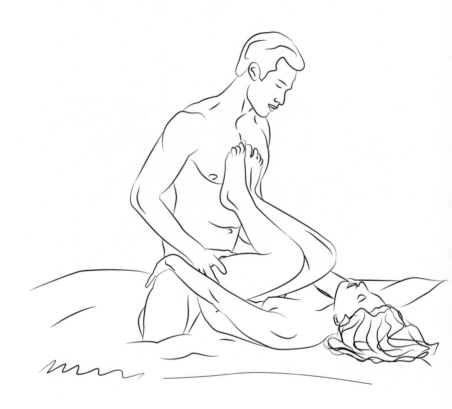

fortable moving in for the win. Instead of stretching her legs out or wrapping her ankles around his head, this simple position just asks that she put her feet flat on his chest. Her goal is to have her big toes touching her big toes and her heels touching her heels. The closer her feet are together, the tighter he will fit inside of her. She can practice flexing her PC muscles so that the tension around his penis will expand and contract, giving him a rhythm to work with as he goes in and out of her. Doing this feels good for him and for her—flexing those muscles helps to build orgasms!

For a penetrating take on a little fancy footwork, this position is a perfect go-to.

Over the Shoulder Ankle Holder

People joke about being able to put their legs over their heads, but it's actually quite a useful skill. For instance . . .

She lies down on the bed, with her legs curled up to her chin. This angle will have her primed and ready for him when he lies down on top of her. Hovering over her, he should help her rest her ankles on

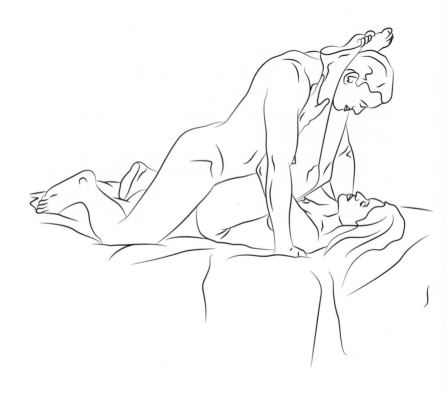

"Be plain in dress, and
sober in your diet;
In short, my deary,
kiss me, and be quiet."

—Lady Mary Wortley Montagu

either side of his shoulders. She can keep her knees bent, so there's no crazy stretching that's required of her beforehand in order to limber up. It's important that her ankles are snugly around his neck, rather than just draping her legs over his shoulders, because the closeness of her feet together also signifies how tightly she'll fit around him inside her.

His weight on top of her will keep her knees close to her chest, which gives him greater depth as he moves in and out of her. This position still allows both partners to maintain eye contact throughout, and even for him to lean down for the occasional passionate kiss. In moments like these, though, he should be careful not to put too much weight on top of her; otherwise her knees will prevent her from breathing easily.

This position gives some kinky legwork an intimate twist!

Leg Lock

You're stuck together, a matching set, just perfect for each other—at least in this position!

She lies down on the edge of the bed with one or both legs raised. He stands in front of her, with one leg firmly on the floor, and the other on the bed for

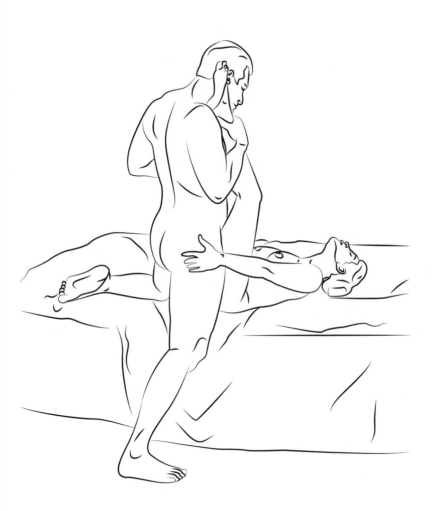

leverage. By holding one of her legs in the air, and the other comfortably to her side, he can enter her deeply. If she's feeling really hot and heavy, she can grab his hips to pull him in deeper as he thrusts. If deep action will get her riled up but not all the way there, she can masturbate while he watches, or he can rub her clitoris as he goes.

BALLET SLIPPER

In no simpler terms, this position is just plain pretty. Like a ballet slipper, it looks beautiful while performing a very important purpose. And luckily for you, this purpose is the kind that gives orgasms, not blisters.

She should arrange herself on all fours, while he kneels upright behind h er. He should raise one leg so that his foot is resting flat on the bed (or floor, roof—wherever). She should raise her leg on the same side back and up, so that her thigh rests on top his, and her calf and foot extend comfortably up and behind him. Using her hips as his guide, he can control his thrusts while she uses her arms in front of her for support. With her leg up high, he'll be able to get more of himself inside her, and she'll get more cli-

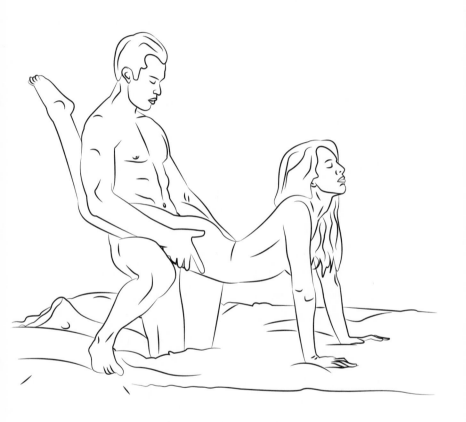

toral stimulation. He can use this angle to cup her breasts, or if he doesn't feel like being gentle, he can tug on her hair a little.

The legwork in this position gives doggie style a whole new aesthetic, and feels pretty excellent in the process.

THE HOME STRETCH

Nothing starts off the day like a good morning stretch, or a good morning sexing. What better way to start off the day than combining the two?!

She lies head first at the edge of the bed. He kneels in front of her, scooting her forward as he inserts himself inside her. The best way to move in to this position is by doing it naturally—she should let out a big stretch, extending her arms off the bed and grazing her fingertips along the floor. The arch of her back should coincide with the curve of the bed's edge, so that way nothing is being strained in the wrong places. He can help her reach the floor by maneuvering her hips, but more importantly, keeping them on the bed so she doesn't fall off. This position gives him a great view of her stomach and chest as she loosens up her body. Since her head is now lower

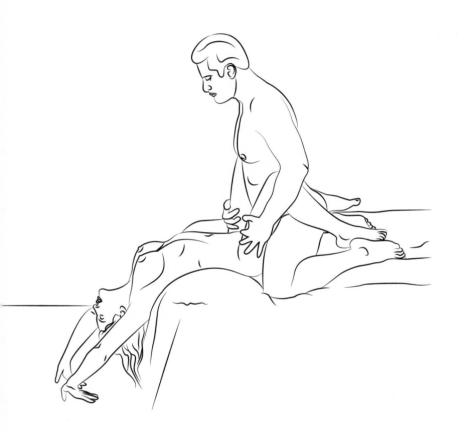

than her core, this good morning tryst will exaggerate her building climax. His positioning right in front of her open hips is also perfect for some deep action.

And of course, there's no need to restrict this position to the morning. Keep stretching all day!

CATCHER'S POSITION

As one of the most important positions in baseball, it's no surprise that the catcher's stance would come in handy on a different playing field.

Pretty much all that is required of him is to lie back and enjoy the view. As he lies down, she should crouch down on top of him, with her knees close to her chest, and her feet flat on the bed. It's not enough to just wriggle around on top and look pretty. She should be using her quad muscles for all they're worth, bringing her whole pelvis up and down his shaft. If she gets tired, she can slow down the pace, hovering over his tip and then let gravity take over—rinse and repeat. The stance of her legs opens her up so that she can go the whole length of his shaft. By leaning back slightly, the tip of his penis will be flush with the inside wall of her vagina, which will feel great for both involved. While she's busy doing all of

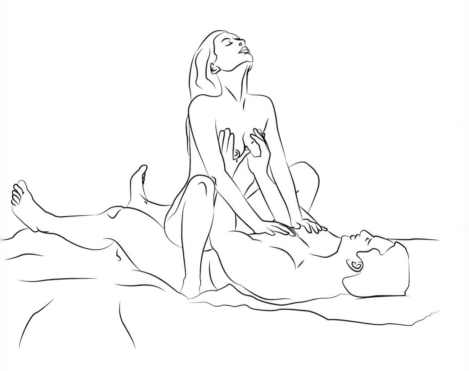

the manual labor, he can make use of his idle hands and massage her breasts, rub her clitoris, or just hold on to her waist for dear life.

Embrace an All-American pastime and score a few runs with her in the hot seat.

Chapter Six

Advanced Placement

INTRODUCTION

These positions are for the over-achievers. You know who you are. Each of these is physically possible, if athletically strenuous. Just a teensy, itty bitty note: For anything that involves lifting your partner, you'll want to watch that you don't drop said partner on his or her head.

If you're naturally just better than everyone at everything, these should be a cinch. For the rest of us, these moves are something to aspire to, fantasize about, and spend hundreds of dollars on Bikram yoga for. But even if you *know* you don't bend that way, give these moves a try, and who knows? Maybe some day you'll be fucking upside down!

THE WILD WALL POSITION

This is for when you've both been very bad—so get up against the wall! You'll both need good balance for this one, and she'll need strong legs to stay up for very long while he bench-presses her from below!

He lies on the floor with his head propped on a pillow and his feet up high against the wall. She

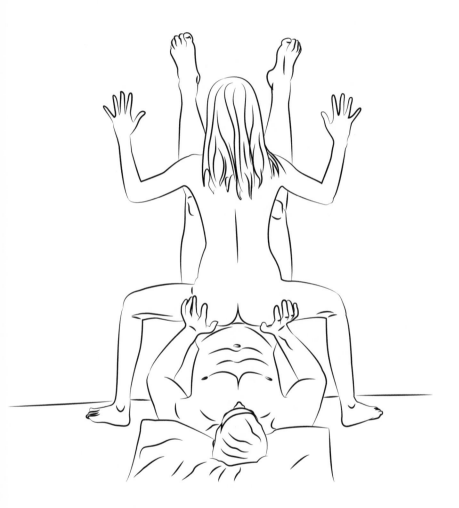

straddles his torso while pressing her body to his legs and her hands against the wall. She can control the speed and depth of their movements by raising and lowering her hips, holding his ankles for traction if she needs to. He can help by supporting her ass with his free hands, but she'll definitely still feel the burn! From down below, he gets a great view of the proceedings, and she gets a workout.

If you can stay up long enough to get in place, you've already won half the battle. But if you can master it, this position gives you a lot of control over thrust speed and depth. If slow and steady wins your race, this is just the position for you to try!

ARC DE TRIOMPHE

This twisty backwards position will wow you—if you can stay up long enough to get it right! This move requires strength and balance, and a lot of flexibility. It takes a good amount of core strength to lower yourself like that, so if you need a hand, you can use props to "walk" down into position.

He stands wide-legged and holds her thighs around his hips as she holds on to his neck. When he is inside her, she slowly lowers herself back until

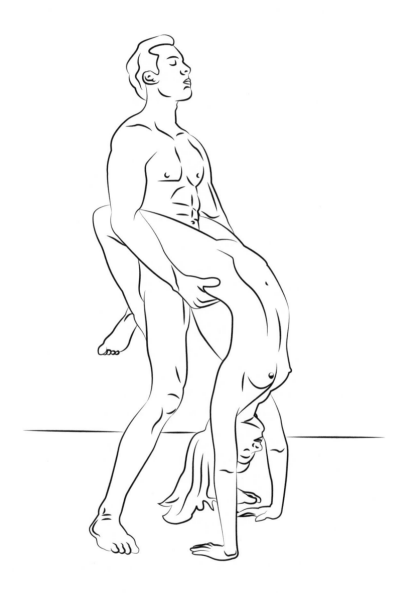

her hands touch the floor. He thrusts into her as she braces herself with her hands on the floor.

Arch your back to try out different angles. You can try this when you're walking down into position, leaning back on the bed or down to a chair.

THE CONTORTIONIST

You won't have to twist into a pretzel for this position, but it might make you twist and shout! It's tricky to do, but a ton of fun. Strong back, shoulders, and core muscles are needed for this move, so be careful if you've been avoiding the gym.

She starts in a push-up position with her thighs on the mattress and her upper body supported by her hands on the floor. He positions himself between her legs, rolls her onto her side, pulling a leg up to his shoulder and supporting her body weight with both hands around her hips.

This sideways position gives you a nice tight fit while you're fighting to stay upright, so it's worth the cost of admission! Since he's got two feet on the ground, he's mostly in control for this move. If you like strong strokes, or a rhythm that gets a little wild, this position is a good option for you. But if you like it a

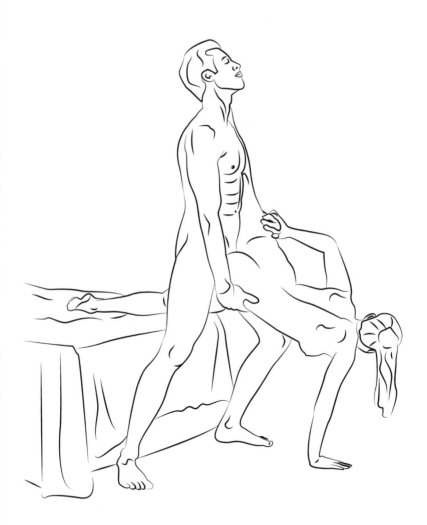

little rough, you may want to tone it down here: if his thrusts get too enthusiastic, he might send her flying!

THE BOBSLED

Also known as "sledding on bob," this position can be fun in any season! This number requires strong core muscles, good balance, and a tight grip (of each other's hands)!

He sits on the edge of a chair. She climbs on top, straddling him and sliding onto his penis. Then, once they're ready, she starts to lean backward and move her legs from his sides to rest on his shoulders. She can hold his hands as she lowers herself backward, which will also keep her from sliding right off his lap.

Once they're in position, she can use her legs to brace herself against him as they both use their handhold for some gravity-fighting friction.

WALK THE PLANK

Pirates are the sexy bad boys of the sea, so grab your naughty seafarer and make him walk your plank!

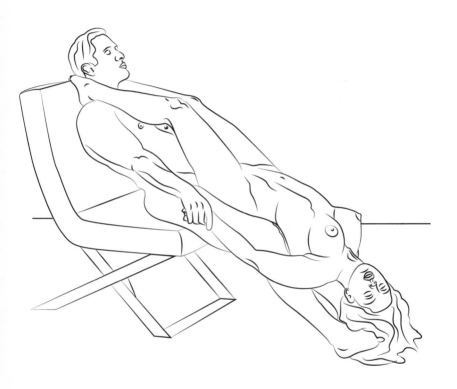

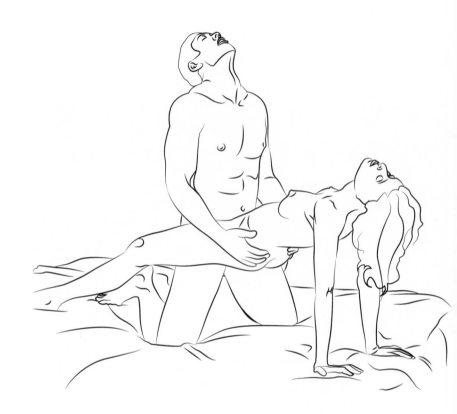

She lies back on the bed with her legs spread. He kneels between her knees and lifts her hips to meet his. She supports her upper body on her hands, in a crabwalk position. As they go, she can rock her legs from straight to bent, and back again to help him thrust their way to paradise. The rocking motion (how apropos for these seafarers!) will help ease the tension in her arms, so that she doesn't get too tired from holding her body weight up. He should be too distracted by the fact that his penis is inside her vagina to notice that his arms hurt from holding her.

This position gives both partners a great view of the coastline! With her torso stretched out, he can watch her boobs get all nice and jiggly as they plunge away, she can admire his upper half, and they both can watch the whole "now you see it, now you don't!" magic show that comes along with thrusting.

NEVER LET ME GO

Hold on tight for this swinging position!

Standing sex can be a challenge, and even if you've got a man of steel on hand for the heavy lifting, the

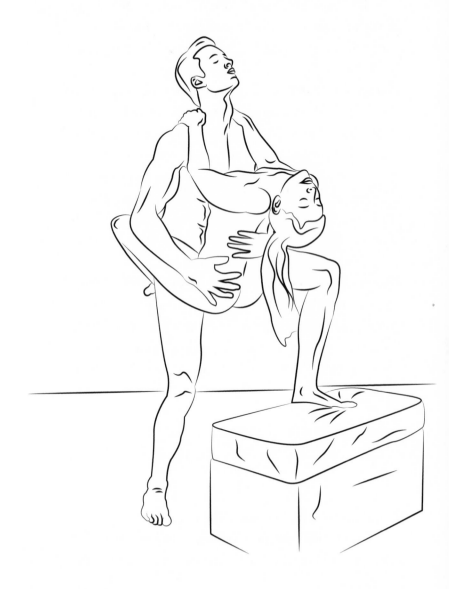

logistics can be limiting. This position gives you the best of standing sex—with a little extra leverage.

He stands with one leg planted on the ground, and the other propped on a sturdy stool or ottoman. She climbs on up, holding his shoulders and wraps her legs around his torso. Once they're moving, she can lean back, with his hand supporting her lower back.

He can use his supporting hands to rub and fondle her ass as she arches her back and leans away: her movements push her hips closer to his, and give them a tighter fit. With this move you'll never want to let go!

THE BEACHCOMBER

Every beach has one—the guy with the headphones and the metal detector, wandering in search of buried treasure. (Seriously, WHERE did he buy that?) For those of us who are less proactive about finding valuables in large piles of sand, and more interested in being naked—this position at least lets you perform your own hunt for treasure.

She places her hands flat on the floor, as if she's doing a push-up. He stands behind her and lifts her

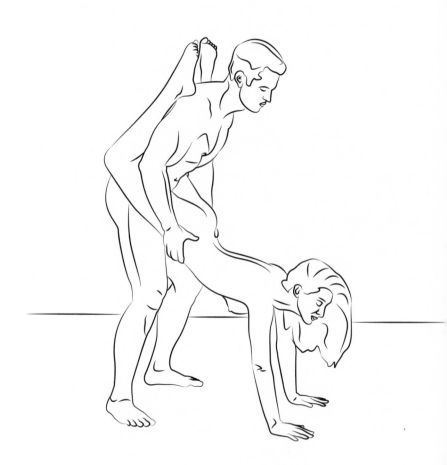

legs, resting her hips on his thighs. Placing a leg on either side of his torso, she curls them up and back so that her heels are comfortably along his shoulder blades. (Her calves and feet should be parallel to his back.) To make this easier on both involved, he should be leaning forward as he holds on to her hips. It's important for her to keep loose and limber during this position. If she's too rigid with her arms locked, he may hurt her back when he thrusts.

Both should be moving together to make this lusty thrust the hottest find on the beach.

FIVE HOT WAYS TO LIMBER UP

Anyone can have good sex, but to have insane acrobatic super sex, you need to be in top physical condition. Being in good shape makes everything a little better: exercise can stave off depression, give you more energy, help you eat better, and even give your car a nice new wax (okay, maybe not that last one). But exercise is boring and completely un-fun, at least in my humble opinion. So I've come up with some options that don't suck so much.

Dance

Any kind of dancing will do. Dancing is an incredible thing: It's art, it's exercise, and it's what your body does automatically whenever someone puts on some groovy tunes. If you want to make dancing part of your exercise routine, you can sign up for classes to learn anything from classic ballet to the very un-classic but trendy pole dancing, or even try belly dancing. If that's not your style there's sure to be a dance class that moves to your kind of music, so check out your local dance schools.

If you'd rather dance with nobody watching, you can pick up some moves through online videos, or with a dance-themed video game. Or you can turn on some music and groove out on your own: don't be embarrassed if you're rocking lame middle school dance moves like the moves aren't so important as long as you're bending, shaking, twisting, shouting and getting the blood pumping while you rock and roll.

Do Stuff Naked

Anyone who's ever gone skinny-dipping knows that being naked makes everything more exciting. Why not bring that to your exercise routine? You might want to keep your naked calisthenics at home, although there are some gyms that welcome naked patrons.

There are some exercises that work better au naturel than do others. Anything with a lot of movement, like running, jumping jacks, or jump rope, can be painful in the nude because it makes your bodacious bits bounce. Not fun or comfortable. Slow moving exercises are great while naked: try doing your stretches, sit-ups, and other core exercises like planks. If you're into yoga, try your usual routine with a naked twist! Spending time naked gives you a chance to get comfortable with your body, which is a necessary ingredient for really good sex! So strip, then give me 20!

Compete

If you're having trouble getting motivated, you might need the extra push of a little competition. This works best with a partner, but so do the positions in this book, so you probably have someone in mind.

You can get your competitive activity by picking up a game of an old standby like basketball, or by racing, either on foot or on a bike. If your competitive strengths are more on the digital side, you can still make a winning streak work for you: make new rules for your video game play to give push-up penalties for in-game losses. You can even make a game of it: make different in-game actions "cost" different exercises. Or you can use a deck of cards to pick a random exercise whenever your character dies: just assign each suit an exercise (for example, hearts are sit-ups, spades are push-ups, diamonds are jumping jacks and clubs are planks), then when you draw a card you do that number of that kind of exercise, so for a six of hearts, you would do six sit-ups!

Kid Stuff

Raid your garage for some fun props to make exercise less lame! There are plenty of things to do that will get your heart pumping, but that don't look like exercise at all! Dig out the Frisbee and set up a one-on-one game, or run around with the soccer ball for a bit. Better yet, pull out your Hula-Hoop and get in shape by gyrating your hips! Grab some chalk and play hopscotch in the driveway, or get the jump rope and show off your double-dutch skills. Find something that makes you want to move, and then stick with it!

Have Hot Sex!

Sex burns calories. Did you know that? Everyone should know: sex isn't just good, it's good for you! Having good sex helps you relieve stress, reduce pain, and get closer with your partner, so when you're getting down and dirty, keep that in mind! Any position can get your blood pumping, but positions that get you moving work even better. The more you're bumping and grinding, the healthier you'll be!

THE TRAPEZE ARTIST

This circus act will turn you topsy-turvy once you master it! It doesn't look like it should work, but if you tilt your head and turn the book upside down, you can see how everything fits together. Both partners need a lot of strength for this position, so you may need to work up to it!

He rests his elbows on a chair or ottoman, extending his legs straight back into a plank. She lies on a pillow on the floor and aligns her naughty bits with his. She then spreads her legs and lifts them up and back over her head, curling up while pressing her palms flat against the floor.

She's bent in half and upside down, so thrusting feels a lot different!

But while you're enjoying your roll in the hay, be conscious of her neck and his lower back, since both are vulnerable in this position.

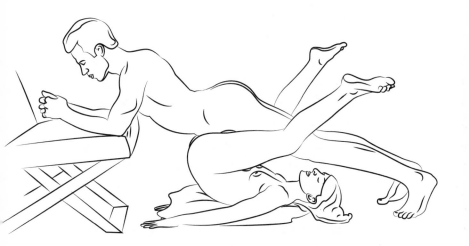

LEANING TOWER

He'll lean your tower of Pisa! This position is like the ultimate trust fall, so don't let go! It requires a lot of strength for him to support her safely, so he better be eating his Wheaties!

She lies on a pillow on the floor. He stands in front of her, facing her, as he pulls her hips up to rest on his thighs with her legs straight out behind him. He should lean over until he is at the right height to slide into her. She stretches so that her body is held straight and stiff (like the old slumber party game, "light as a feather, stiff as a board," if she stays rigid, it is a lot easier for him to hold her up!). She can hold on to his calves for more support, as he thrusts down and forward.

This position may tire her out quickly (or give her a neck ache) but it's so fun while it lasts! Keep strokes slow and deep to make good use of this angled position and enjoy the tight new sensations.

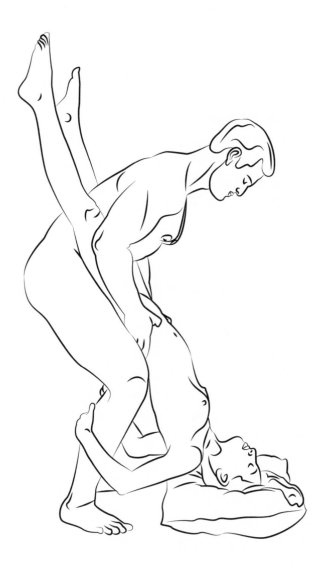

BRIDGE TO PARADISE

Show off your moves with this visually stimulating oral position. The challenge is to stay up while he rocks your world!

She plays it old school like 5th period gym class, and poses on the floor in a classic "bridge" position. He kneels between her legs and holds her thighs for more support. See how close to paradise you can get before your bridge comes falling down!

CANNON BALL

Imagine he's preparing for takeoff: Powering up into the air takes coordination, some serious thigh strength, and a nice lift from her booster.

She lies on a pillow on the floor, bent into a pike position (legs bent at the hip, aimed above and past her head). He stands at her bottom, facing away from her, and lowers himself in while pushing back and down on her thighs.

This creative configuration gets her a rarely seen view of his nice butt, and him a good amount of control over his thrusts. If she starts to slide off the pillow, she can grip his ankles for traction.

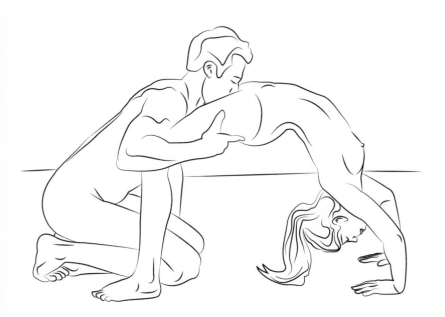

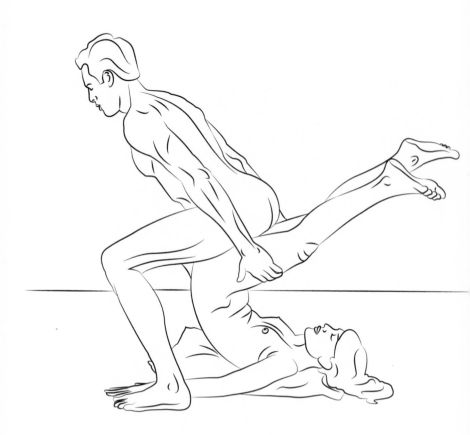

"True beauty dwells
in deep retreats,
Whose veil is unremoved
Till heart with heart
in concord beats,
And the lover is beloved."

—William Wordsworth

FIVE MORE WAYS TO PLAY: HOT ORAL POSITIONS TO TRY

Looking for even more fun positions to try? Here are five more conjugal configurations that will blow you away. Try these hot oral positions and see if you don't find a new favorite way to go down!

Over Easy

None of this 69 bullshit, you want his attention front and center when he's going down. With him focused on you, you can tell him exactly what you want—or, since he has a front-row seat, you can show him!

He lies on the bed. She climbs on top and straddles his head, supporting her upper body with her arms above his head. His hands are free to roam around her pleasure center, to spank her ass, or to reach up and tweak her nipples. She has her hands free to hold on to the headboard and holler when he hits the right spot.

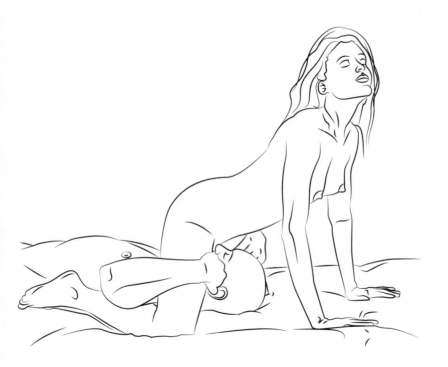

Since she's on top, she has control over the angle and depth of his strokes. She can tilt her hips to adjust the angle of his approach, or to show him where she needs a little more TLC. Since all of his attention is on her, she can call out instructions, and tell him what she wants.

The Lounge

Got a crick in your neck? This is a great position to shake up your blow-job moves, and it's got everything going for it. He lies on the bed on his side in the classic "lounge" position. She kneels on the floor beside the bed with her torso resting on the bed (if your bed is high off the ground, try this on the couch!). She loops her arm over his bottom knee to pull his hips closer to her.

At this angle she has two free hands and full access to his penis, balls, and ass. Not only that, but she has tons of possible angles for fellatio: she can slide him into her mouth sideways for a spicy new feel, or with a slight reposition, she can take him in the more traditional front-entry position, or slide down the bed and approach from below, kissing

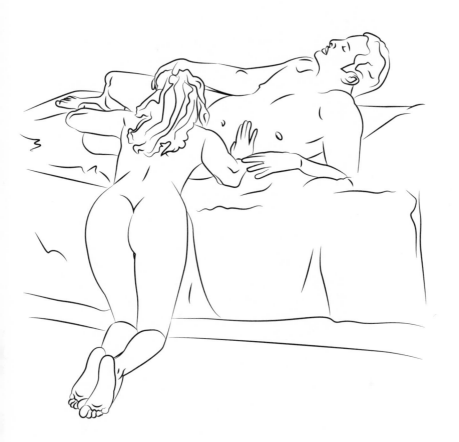

and caressing him as he watches. From his vantage point he has a front row seat, and since he's comfortably reclined, he has his hands free to guide her right where he wants her. Remember that the trick to comfortable oral sex is changing positions before you get sore, so if you're bored, switch it up and see how he likes it when you try something new!

The Wallflower

This position will have her blooming in no time—but you'd better work fast, because this balancing act is trickier than it looks!

She stands with her back against the wall. He sits cross-legged and scoots up to the wall to face her. She lifts one leg and drapes it over his shoulder while he moves his head between her legs.

With her leg over his shoulder, she can pull him closer as he works his magic, and he can get a thrill from having her pushed up against the wall. He's got access to all her sexy bits, so he can use his hands while his mouth is busy. This position is a lot like a traditional blow job: the receiving party gets to stand and watch as her partner goes down on her. Just

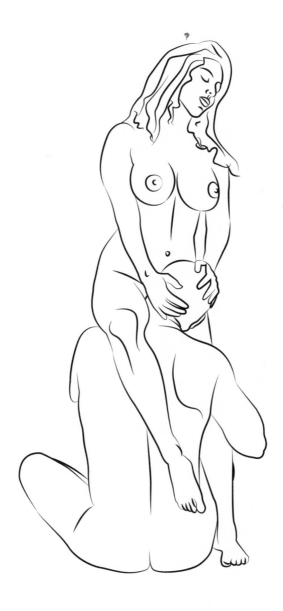

like with those blow jobs, her hand on his head helps her tell him when she wants more. It's a powerful vantage point, with a hot view!

Tonsil Hockey

How do you feel about deep throat? If you're looking for a position that gives you the deepest fit, you've found it. Seriously, this position is like the deep sea drilling of the sex world. You'll end up going all the way to China. It's a deep throat position, is what I'm saying.

The positioning is simple. She lays face up on the bed with her head just hanging off the edge. He stands by the edge of the bed, facing her. As they get into position, he holds onto her torso so she doesn't slide off the bed, and she wraps her arms around his legs to pull them closer.

If she's a blow job beginner, this move is not for you, unless you both like a lot of choking and sputtering to your sex. On the bottom, she doesn't have a lot of control over how fast or deep he goes. But if she's up for it, this move gives her access to all of him!

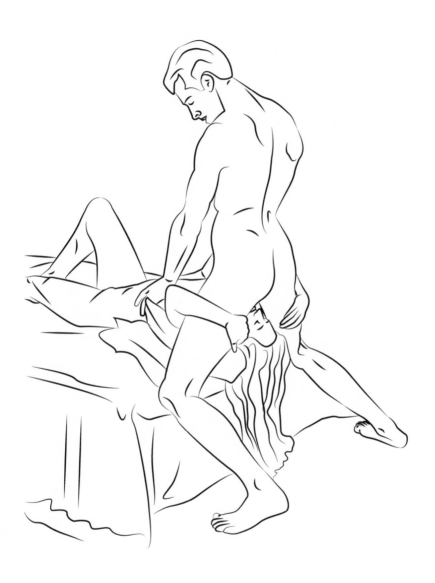

Mission Control

Guide him to landing pad and show him how it's done! This position lets her be in full control of the fun as he goes down.

She kneels on the bed and sits back on her heels. He crouches on the bed, facing her, as she guides him toward her sexy bits. This move focuses the attention of the star of her show: the clitoris! Having her knees drawn up in that position makes it hard for him to face-plant (Note to guys: Can you stop doing this? And no motorboating down there, either: a girl wants a touch of finesse!), and gives her a chance to show him how she really wants it. Have him change up his movements, going from fast to slow and back again!

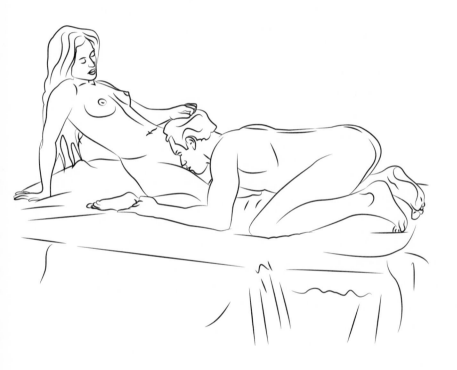

OTHER SMUT
BY MARISA BENNETT

Fifty Shades of Pleasure: A Bedside Companion:
Sex Secrets that Hurt So Good

Surrender to Your Desire for Naughty
Bedroom Pleasures . . .

If hot erotic romance novels have had you fantasizing about certain naughty pleasures, or if you just want to add a little spice to your sexy love sessions, this kinky how-to will bring your fantasies to life. Explore the pleasure of a little pain, flex muscles you didn't know you had through hot sex positions, and learn how to make or break the rules in your playtime romp.

With a light, playful tone, this book eases you into the stingingly sweet side of sex. Each section features excerpts from the Kama Sutra or classic erotica, extra tips like "Dirty Talk Dos and Don'ts," and offers further resources to continue your naughty education. Gather your ben wa balls and feather ticklers while this handbook gives you the rundown on all the hot moves you've been wanting to try, from beginner bondage techniques and starter spanking to hot wax and flogging—no dungeon required!

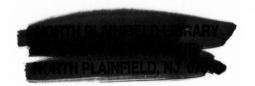